FRESH OUT OF EMT SCHOOL

TIPS AND TRICKS FOR THE NEW EMT

ALBERT REYES

STEVEN WATTS

PUBLISHED BY FASTPENCIL PUBLISHING

First Edition

Copyright © Albert Reyes 2017

http://fp.fastpencil.com

Printed in the United States of America

TABLE OF CONTENTS

ACKNOWLEDGMENT

I would like you thank God for saving me and allowing me to go back to EMT school.

Also to Victory Outreach Church for taking me in and providing a home where I could get my life together. To the Pastors and leadership which are too numerous to add here. But a special thank you to Pastor Ed and Mitzi who showed me how to be a man of God.

My wife Lucy for always wanting me to be the best, my children Victoria, Soraya, and Cyrus who drive me to be a better Father every day

Ignacio and Tiffany Garcia, Rachel Zepeda, Jackie Hua, Delfino Romayor, and, Steve Watts for helping me put this book together.

Tom Sanchez, John Sagli, Joe English, Garrick Ongolea, Sue Stapleton, Samantha Burch and Johnny Reyes who read my book and inspired me to go forward with this project.

For all my Paramedic friends who gave their "Words of Wisdom". Thank you for believing in me and contributing your years of experience.

Thank you all so much.

PREFACE

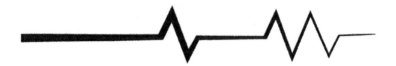

The birth of this book started when I came to work one day and spotted this young kid fresh out of EMT school. He was one of the nicest kids I ever met. It was his first day and he was smiling, happy and excited to be there. After a half hour of standing there and not knowing what to do, I began to sense the anxiety within him. I began to sense his fear and uncertainty. It reminded me of my first day not really knowing anybody... thinking, can I really do this without messing everything up? People's lives would be in my hands, could I really do this job? Where do I start? School had prepared me but I knew there would be so much more to learn. Most importantly, I would have a field training officer that would either say I failed or succeeded. I remember grabbing the young man by the shoulder and saying, "Do you know what to do right now?" He looked at me with a sense of relief and said, "No". I began to take this young man to the side and show him the ropes. I also prepared him for his first day; what he could expect, some tips and tricks and what to do at that very moment. I gave him a sense of direction and I could tell the young man was very grateful. From that day on I knew I had to write something for these new EMT's. I had to help them...

INTRODUCTION

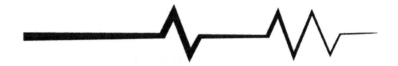

    My name is Albert Reyes and I've been an EMT for the past 16 years. For seven of those years, I was also a FTO (Field Training Officer). I currently work on an ambulance in Santa Clara County, California. I wrote this book to help new EMT's make a smooth transition into EMS. To give you a heads up, the inside scoop, and just plain tips and tricks of the trade–information that will help you stand out and shine above other new EMT's.

    This book is not an EMT course! It will not help you pass EMT school, show you how to be an EMT, or describe how to assess a patient. That's what school is for. This book is designed to help you transition into the field once you get hired on an ambulance. I have gained all my experience by working on an ambulance–many nights, days, and hours on an ambulance. Experienced EMT's can benefit from this book, but this book is for brand new EMT's. This book is geared towards working in the 911 system. Stay tuned for the next book in this series FRESH OUT OF EMT SCHOOL called "BLS LIFE." It will focus on working in the BLS system.

Beginning a career in EMS can be stressful, challenging, and even scary. I will be giving you a lot of information in this book about your role in the 911 system. Fresh Out of EMT School will primarily benefit EMT-B's that will be assisting AEMT's or Paramedics. It is meant to teach and give the EMT-B their roles when assisting the person with the highest level of care on scene. My hope is to challenge you, not to scare you. I will not share horror stories or traumatic events. You will develop your own experiences. It's inevitable on the 911 system. 85% of your calls will not be an emergency. In fact, most of your calls will be helping people in a different way. While you will have your share of saving lives, most of the time you will be helping people with your smile, gentle care, empathy, compassion and sometimes just holding their hands. My experience as a new EMT was pretty exciting and scary all at the same time. When you are a new EMT you have to remember you are just that—new, ripe, and fresh out of school. What we do in the field is sometimes very different than what we learn in EMT school. When you're new, you will be treated as such. Earning respect comes with a great attitude, an open mind, and old-fashioned hard work. Your effort will show how bad you want to work in EMS. My hope is to relieve you from some of the stress and anxiety that can come with being new.

Pay attention in class because you will need to have the basic EMT knowledge and skills. That is a must. There is nothing worse than having to teach an EMT the basics all over again. Being a hard worker and knowing your basic EMT knowledge will at least let FTOs know that you have the basics down, and they can work with you on the rest. Again, they don't want to go over fundamentals with you—you should know it already. I can't stress that enough.

You will be new and there is nothing you can do about it. Don't try to act like something you're not and pretend you know everything. Anybody in the field who has been doing this for awhile can tell you are new. Accept it and be willing to learn and grow. Start your EMS career with a great attitude and you will do well. My hope is that you will read this book and feel comfortable on your first day of work. That you will go in confident (not cocky) and take on the challenge of being a great EMT. I hope to inspire you to take this challenge head on.

<u>*"Tips and Tricks for the new EMT"*</u>
A good EMT is like the Medic's Surgical Assistant, always paying attention and

handing equipment before the Medic has to ask for it.

FRESH OUT OF EMT SCHOOL... WHAT TO DO NOW?

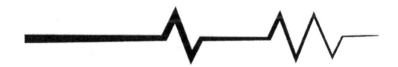

HOW TO START

So you're fresh out of school and now you want a job. Good. Getting your EMT certification will open up many doors for your life! All of my experience will come from working on an ambulance, but there are numerous jobs EMT's can do. They can work in the Fire Service (most firefighters are EMT's), in a hospital as an ER Tech, at an amusement park or sporting event – the list goes on and on. So get going.

- EMT's are in high demand so start searching in your area.

- Start doing ride-alongs or volunteering wherever you can, on an ambulance or with your local Fire Dept. It all looks good on your resume and in your interview.

Get ready for that National Registry Test. There are many books to help you study for that. Go to emtb.com, cram.com or quizlet.com and search for EMT National Registry.

APPLY NOW

The fear of not being hired stops most people from even applying. Don't believe it. Go and apply at your county ambulance provider. Most of you will want to work 911 right away but BLS (Basic Life Support) is where most EMT's start off. Don't let BLS scare you away.

BLS does not respond to 911 calls but can be called on when ambulance levels are low in the county. BLS will mostly do inter-facility transports, long distance transports, appointments, courthouse standbys, sports standbys, etc. They are sometimes more busier than ALS and will help you gain a lot of experience before transferring to an ALS system.

One of the myths is that they are not hiring right now. I've seen so many people not apply because they heard that they are not hiring. Go and apply for yourself and let them tell you they are not hiring. In EMS you will also have to knock on doors more than once. Apply again and again.

Don't worry about bugging them. Sometimes persistence pays off. Be determined!

People will tell you that you need this and that to get hired. That they are only looking for medics, you need to speak a foreign language, etc. Go and apply. Apply everywhere. You may not get the first EMS job you apply for—it's ok. You will gain experience while you are waiting to get hired at your dream job, and that experience will eventually help you get where you want to be. Remember, companies will hire somebody with experience over somebody who has none. You may have to work BLS for a while. I worked on Basic Life Support, Critical Care Transports, Neonatal Intensive Care Unit, Pediatric Intensive Care Unit transports, Lifelight transports, and ALS inter-facility transports. Put your time and work in. It's worth it.

RIDE ALONGS/VOLUNTEER IN ER

Go prepared. Always do research and have questions ready to ask when the moment comes. Have necessary equipment on you to do your basic EMT skills. Dress to impress. Iron your clothes, shine your boots, and tuck in your shirt. There's nothing worse than a sloppy looking EMT. Smile and meet as many people as possible. You never know who will be on your interview panel as you are getting hired. Your attitude should show some humility and an eagerness to learn. Be respectful and listen to directions. Bring a notepad and take notes. Get in there and do some patient care. Don't wait for them to tell you your job. Get your hands dirty!

THE OFFERING

What I'm going to tell you right here is going to score you major points. When doing ride-alongs or volunteering in an ER, know that everybody in EMS loves FOOD, COFFEE, AND SWEETS! Do not come empty handed! Make sure you bring an "Offering" of your appreciation. Gift cards and thank you cards are greatly appreciated. Just don't come empty handed. This will probably be free for you so come prepared and share a small token of your gratitude for this experience.

THE INTERVIEW

Again, dress to impress. Shave and make sure you smell good. Use proper language. I used to sit on interview panels, and wearing a suit shows professionalism. It won't disguise your attitude and heart but it sure makes you look good. It is a must. Show them that you are serious about EMS and professionalism. Don't forget to give a nice firm handshake and make eye contact with everyone in the room. The first handshake will often make or break you because it is the interviewer's first impression of you. It starts there in the interview room. Do mock interviews with friends, coworkers, and family. Everything helps.

Go prepared by studying beforehand. Read some books on going through an interview. You should have an answer for every question. Be familiar with what questions they might be asking you. Find somebody that went through the process. Ask them what questions they were asked and what you should be prepared for. Most interviews will start off with a question related to "Tell us about yourself." Be able to give the panel an inside look of you personally and professionally. Most interviews will also have scenario questions about patient care or scene safety. One of the most important questions will come at the end with, "Do you have anything to add?" Have a summative "speech" prepared explaining why you are a good fit for the position and don't forget to thank the panelists for their time. Be prepared to take a written or skills test right on the spot. Brush up on your assessments, scope of practice, and anatomy/physiology. Be prepared for anything.

WORDS FROM THE WISE; PROVERBS FROM TODAY'S PARAMEDICS

"I think I would tell that new EMT what I tell all the new people... There are no certainties in EMS. Recognize how important the job is, don't cut corners, form good habits. Work hard, sleep harder, love your job, and don't be influenced by those who are burnt out. You only get one chance at this job, make it count, because when you're 80 years old, you're going to look back and realize that you're never going to be this awesome ever again."

– John McNulty (EMT / Paramedic) 12 years experience.

"First day...this is a job for people with a servant's heart. If you got into the field thinking it was an extended episode of Rescue Me or Chicago Fire, then you will surely be disappointed. Less than 10% of our calls require the critical skills and lifesaving interventions that we're trained for. Book knowledge is critical, but a balance of experience and education is required. Listen to those with experience, more than likely they've been in your situation before. This is a team sport. A collective effort is required. No one runs a call without help. If you think you've learned and seen it all...it's

time to find another career. A good EMT anticipates his/her partner's next move. Always think ahead. If you have a question, ASK! No one knows it all"
— **Jason Leech (Fire Fighter Paramedic) 23 years experience.**

"Whatever you do, in an emergency, if you are not in danger, please do not run! Walk with a purpose but don't run. And always wash your hands after you touch a patient!"
— **Florin Florea (Fire Fighter Paramedic) 18 years experience.**

"I have two important things I tell all new partners EMT's or paramedics...
First, if you're new in this county and you're not sure where you are or where a hospital is, ask me before you leave the scene. It's easier for me to give you directions before we're lost and I can't tell where we are. Second, when we're on scene always be within my vision. If poop hits the fan and we need to bail out, I don't have to look for you. We're a team, you and I are it and I need to know if I can count on you to be there for me and vice versa, even if other responders are with us".
— **Zia Warda (EMT / Paramedic) 26 years experience.**

"My words of wisdom....every day, do the best you can, in the time you have, at the moment you're in. Meaning each day is important, and each day is different because of experiences, time, and learning from others whom you work with or care for. The wisdom comes from hard work at being prepared for the events of your patients' worst moments of their lives."
– Jim Howard (EMT / Paramedic) 27 years experience.

"You know, I'm pretty chill and don't expect too much from my EMT. I know it's scary, so I don't pressure them much, but if I have to answer the question, I would have to say obviously know your stuff and if not then ask. I hate EMT's who don't know and try to wing it. Like direction or using the equipment. But I like an EMT who's not lazy...set me up ready for the next call. Like putting the patches on 12 leads, set IV up, or saline lock. Not being lazy at least shows me they're trying and working hard. Also getting a facesheet helps. I hate having to get it after doing my EPCR."
– Anthony Nguyen (EMT / Paramedic) 17 years experience.

FTO TIME AND YOUR FIRST DAY

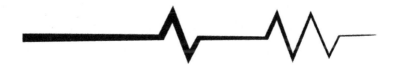

FTO TIME (Field Training Officer)

FTO time is a very crucial time to focus. It will make or break you. Look at it as a tryout. The FTO has the authority to say you fit or don't fit. This is a time to prove yourself. You want to show your FTO that you can take full ownership on scene with a patient. FTOs will not clear you until they feel they can trust you when you're under pressure. This book will help you come into your training confident but humble. Remember to stay professional at all times. Remember failure to prepare is preparing to fail. Remember that it may seem like a lot in the beginning, but it gets easier as time goes by.

Your FTO is responsible for making sure you are safe, can provide adequate care to patients and understand company policies. They are re-sponsible for your training and evaluation process. Your FTO time can be as long as 4 to 18 weeks. They could be grumpy and mean or happy and nice. It should not matter. If you work hard you will be fine.

When coming in for your first day of FTO time, remember you are invading a partnership for the day. This is their office. Some will treat you as a guest, but others will treat you as a burden, so go in prepared. First things first, don't be late! Arriving on time is late. Twenty to thirty minutes early is on time. Being late will definitely get you started off on the wrong foot. Keep in mind you will be relieving an off-going crew most times and arriving early is greatly appreciated. Make sure you bring a meal. There may not be any time to stop and get something to eat, depending on how busy your county is. Bring a lunch pail with plenty of snacks and water. Again, don't come empty-handed—bring something for the crew. As an initial show of gratitude this is appropriate. But don't be suckered into buying the crew coffee every day as this will become a financial burden. Some will try, so be aware.

APPEARANCE

As mentioned before, come looking sharp and RFA (ready for action) with all the proper equipment you will need on calls. Always have your boots zipped up and your shirts tucked in. Nothing is better than a good looking EMT. Shine your boots, iron your clothes, and take a shower. I know I shouldn't have to tell people this but this is a reality. Some people don't have the same hygiene values as others. You will be working closely with others for a minimum of 12 hours and sitting very closely with other crew members. If I have to sit so long with someone who doesn't shower or have good hygiene, it makes the day unpleasant. Breath mints and gum are huge.

"Tips and Tricks for the new EMT"
Keep a mint or two in your pocket at all times for that morning breath!! At 3am in the morning you'll be in close proximity to your patients. Don't give them another complaint or make them more sick! Bring some for the ambulance too. Ambulance gum is community gum which is for everybody.

Always restock for coming crews. If you happen to leave your new pack of gum or mints, don't expect to get it back full!

" Tips and Tricks for the new EMT"
Never take off a dirty glove, just put a

new one over it. Sweaty hands will make switching gloves impossible!

EQUIPMENT

The minimum amount of equipment you should have on you is disposable gloves (carry a handful in your pocket), safety glasses, stethoscope, scissors (heavy duty shears preferably), pen light, pen, and two-inch tape for taking down information on patients.

"Tips and Tricks for the new EMT"
Always carry 2 pens with you at all times. Cops, EMS personnel, and Firefighters love to borrow pens permanently. You won't get them back!

Miscellaneous Equipment:

Extra pen: for gathering patients' info (meds, medical history, allergies, vital signs, etc.)

Flashlight: very useful when working nights. Maneuvering the gurney in the dark can be tricky.

Face mask: for shielding yourself from airborne and liquid hazards (blood, vomit, saliva, urine, etc.)

Two-inch tape: when you are new this will save you. Attach to your pant leg. You may stand out as the new guy, but who cares? On a critical call you will be moving fast. You will want to give the hospital vital info. Writing on your gloves will eventually get you into trouble—you will eventually throw them away along with all the important information. Do not get into the front of the cab with dirty gloves or you will contaminate that space!

Transpore or clear plastic tape: this is a transparent breathable and perforated plastic medical tape that gives strong adhesion. It is easy to tear and is easy to use with gloves on.

> *"Tips and Tricks for the new EMT"*
> *Fold over the end of the tape after you use a piece. This saves a lot of time for your medic when they are trying to tear off a piece.*

Heavy duty shears: your company-issued shears will not get the job done on tough materials like leather or denim. Removing these items is a must on major trauma calls.

Fanny pack: worn around your waist to hold miscellaneous equipment.

Radio holder: you must carry a radio on you at all times. You will need contact with your dispatch center at all times.

> *"Tips and Tricks for the new EMT "*
> *Always carry a radio on you since you have to be in constant communication with your dispatch. They have to know you are ok. They will run a welfare check on you, meaning the advisement of your status and safety.*

Multi tool or Leatherman: provides numerous miscellaneous tools on scene such as an O2 wrench, window punch, knife, screwdriver, pliers, etc.

Vicks: for sensitive noses. You will face the inevitable smelly call!!! Vicks will save you!!! Pack your nose and approach the scene with caution. There are other alternatives so go with what works for you but have something available. There's nothing worse than the crew on scene laughing at you because you're throwing up!!

Thermals or extra clothes: Some calls take hours of standing on scene. You might be standing in the cold for a very long time. Bring extra clothes or rain gear. It is a terrible feeling being wet and cold all shift.

GETTING FAMILIAR WITH THE AMBULANCE

Remember; get to your shift early!!! A half hour early is on time! Find out where your deployment area is and try to get equipment and keys. Make sure you have the proper safety equipment (helmets, safety vests, high visibility safety gear, etc.) your county requires. Getting there early will allow you to see what condition the ambulance is in. If it's dirty find out where you can wash it and get started.

After washing the rig, jump inside and have a look at where you will be working for the day. Get familiar with each compartment in the back of the ambulance. Find out what is stored and where it is stored. On calls you will immediately want to know where all equipment is—on the ambulance and in your jump bags. Your medic will be depending on you in a critical situation to know where all the equipment is. At the minimum you should know where the BLS equipment is stored. You will eventually learn the ALS equipment.

"Tips and tricks for the new EMT"
When washing the ambulance, try using a window squeegee to get the water off

the flat surfaces on the sides of the rig.
It works better and requires less labor.

When you first get to the inside of your ambulance wipe everything down! You don't know the cleanliness of the crew that was there before you, or what types of germs or sicknesses have been spread to the entire ambulance. Your company should provide you with an antibacterial disinfectant, so wipe everything down that can be wiped down.

"Tips and tricks for the new EMT"
Your company should provide you with
a checklist of every piece of equipment
that needs to be on the ambulance, usu-
ally county mandated.

Check O2 levels and the suction device. Most equipment will have extra pieces that should be attached or close by. For example, your suction canister should have tubing and suction tips (rigid and non-rigid). Suction equipment should be attached somewhere on the suction canister. Check EKG Monitor and the AED for proper function and make sure they are charged. If they require a pre-check then do that. Check all fluid levels under the hood (oil, water, transmission fluid, etc.). Make sure there is gas in your unit. Check the tires and make sure they are filled.

> *"Tips and Tricks for the new EMT"*
> **When getting your ambulance ready to go in service, there are pre-setups that can help Paramedic interventions go more efficiently. Ask your medic to show you how to Spike a Bag!!! Warm IV bags: toss up on dash with heater full blast for those hypothermic patients. IV kits for your medics are a big help. You can wrap up these pieces of equipment into a chux: 2 or 3 IV catheters (different sizes), alcohol preps, tourniquets, 4x4's, and disposable sharps container. Roll these up in a chux and tie up with tourniquet. When your medic is ready to start an IV, BOOM!! He or she doesn't have to go finding every piece need-ed...it's all there.**

Go to the cab of your ambulance and get famil-iar with lights and sirens. Turn them on and make sure they all work. Find out where all the buttons are located and what they are used for. Never be afraid to ask what your equipment does. Locate the radio and familiarize yourself with how you will be communicating with your dispatch.

> *"Tips and Tricks for the new EMT"*
> *You can help your paramedic out by checking expiration dates on medications. While you're doing this, ask questions on how these drugs work. Ask how and what equipment is needed to set up for patient administration.*

Go outside and familiarize yourself with the outside compartments. Most extrication devices will be located in these. Locate backboards, stair chairs, carry alls, and any other devices you will use to extricate patients to the gurney and into the ambulance. Most compartments will also carry road hazard equipment like fire extinguishers, flares, and cleaning equipment.

> *"Tips and Tricks for the new EMT"*
> *Exercise and stretch regularly. Ask anybody in EMS and he or she will tell you to take care of your back! We carry a lot of people around and lift a lot of gurneys. Stay in shape.*

The last thing you should check, which will be one of the most important pieces of your equipment, is the gurney. You will become one with the gurney!!! Continue on to the next chapter to see why.

> *"Tips and Tricks for the new EMT"*
> *For the new EMT, practice, practice, practice your C-Spine skills! In the heat of the moment this skill will come in handy!*

WORDS FROM THE WISE; PROVERBS FROM TODAY'S PARAMEDICS

"Most important thing to be familiar/experienced with as first day EMT—hospital locations. KNOW WHERE YOU ARE GOING when your senior partner can't be up there to show you. Before your first official day, get in your car and drive around the county or district and practice getting to the hospitals from major highways, intersections, or roadways. Put some time in and get comfortable with your surroundings—nothing ticks off your grumpy, old medic partner more than taking 20 minutes to get to a hospital 2.5 miles away! It's important to listen, observe, and take constructive criticism from those who know, have seen it all, and have been where you are now. This is no time for pride or ego; you gotta pay your dues, just like we all did."

– **Kevin Thompson (EMT / Paramedic) 12years experience**.

"If you're stepping onto the rig with me and it is your first day, PLEASE tell me. Tell me if you're unfamiliar with something, you don't understand how something gets put together. I'm more than happy to walk you through it and to help you piece together whatever information you don't have so that you can be successful not only for yourself, but also for me and the people that we serve. I am more than happy and willing to teach anybody that asks. No ego, no judgment, it is a completely different world, that's cool. If you can tell that somebody just doesn't look good, then you automatically know the direction that we are going. Do they need high-flow oxygen? Do you know that I'm going to need a 12-lead or an IV setup? If they look big sick it's probably a pretty good guess that they are. If you aren't sure, you can always ask. Does this guy look sick? And you'll get a nod from me if they are. Remember that all of us were you at some point. Whether the paramedic will admit it or not. We were all new, green, and shaking in our boots before our first day. This is a dog-eat-dog business with a lot of alpha people and assertive personalities. Keep your head down, ask questions, and don't worry if you don't get everything perfectly. Remember, if every choice you make is in the patient's best interest, you can never be wrong.

– Dominic Curcuruto (EMT / Paramedic) 5years experience.

"Get to know the equipment and where everything is on the rig...So when your medic asks you to get something you know exactly where it is. It takes time but I was always thinking two or three steps ahead of my medic. Anything that I can do to make my medic's job easier, I would do. Perfect example if we go on a hypoglycemic patient, I'm already going to be getting the glucose meter prepped up and IV set up with a bag. Also get that Amp of D50 ready for my medic. Always be proactive...always look for something to do. You shouldn't be standing around."

– Daniel Hernandez (EMT / Paramedic) 11 years experience.

"First impression goes a long way. I know it will be intimidating the first day being an EMT. Showing up on time and coming with a good attitude goes a long way for me and having a willingness to learn. I don't mind them asking questions about how to be a good partner and EMT. I was in the same boat 20-plus years ago. The best advice would be treat everyone like it's your own family member—with respect. Throughout my career, I've seen medics, even EMT's, disrespect patients who are at their lows. And that doesn't slide with me cuz that's somebody's father/mother/etc. Treat people right and you'll be rewarded."

– **Darrell Poblete (Fire Fighter / Paramedic) 22 years experience.**

"I remember being really worried about getting lost. I think the best EMT's always get you to the hospital safely. When you're a new EMT you probably think you need to know medical skills or assessments to be a good EMT, but really we just need someone who can push a gurney safely and drive safely to the hospital without getting lost. Knowing how to talk on the radio helps too. I remember having my own county map with all the hospitals marked for a quick reference."

– **Zach Clark (Fire Fighter / Paramedic) 9 years experience.**

"One thing I tell new people is to have big ears and a small mouth. That way they listen and don't talk much. I also tell them to treat everyone like you would want your family to be treated. And treat everyone nice, people in uniform or not, as you never know who they might be. Also when someone is showing or teaching you something that you may already know, don't say you know it already, just listen as you may learn something new or different. Work hard and always be the first to step up to help."

– Eddie Rocha (Fire Fighter / Paramedic) 16 years experience.

"My biggest advice on the first day would just to be to greet people with a smile, be open to what you are going to learn, and be willing to help out in any way. Also to not be afraid to ask questions when you don't know something. Most people in our profession respect that and want to teach. Also to not be discouraged if you have a bad experience or make a mistake and to use it as a learning process. Making mistakes is when you learn the most."
– Jennifer Sims (EMT / Paramedic) 13 years experience.

"#1) Communicate with your partner, no matter what you're thinking, if you're scared, excited, nervous, whatever it is. This is the only way your partner can help you.

#2) Slow the f*** down! Don't drive like an idiot! No more than 10 mph over the speed limit and come close to stopping at red lights. Otherwise I'll want to get you fired. I don't need the added stress of worrying about my partner killing me."
– Don Messamer (EMT / Paramedic) 27 years experience.

"Communication is such an important part of this job. I would like a new EMT to have good communication skills and the ability to interact comfortably with new people. There is a lot of depth and complexity to this job. Basic skills are needed to get your license, but even EMT's and paramedics with 10 years of experience can learn something new. From your first day onward, cultivate an attitude of humility and the desire to learn. If you think you know it all, you're wrong, and you're setting yourself up for trouble."

– Nate Barmore (EMT / Paramedic) 10 years experience.

"First off, be humble but confident. Know your limitations and if you have weaknesses then be open and share them if asked. If you are not familiar with the area then let me know so I can help you get to the hospital. This is very important for Code 3 returns. We all know how exciting it is to be driving with lights and sirens on but a paramedic being tossed around in the back is an ineffective one. Driving 5 to 10 miles over the speed limit is ok but be easy on the brakes. Be an effective listener and if you are not sure what you are doing then ask for help! No matter how crazy the call is, at the end of the day we want to go to our families. Safety is the key."

– Gil Cocio (EMT / Paramedic) 22 years experience.

THE GURNEY

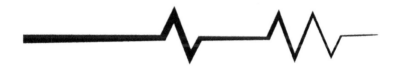

The gurney is one of the most important pieces of equipment you will use and be responsible for. Without a working gurney you will not be able to transport the patient in a safe and efficient way. You will be spending a lot of time with it so get familiar with it right away. Familiarize yourself with all of the moving parts and ensure they work appropriately. Make sure that it is clean, with no old blood or fluids.

Your company will go over proper techniques and safety issues with your gurney. Don't be afraid of it. Start by taking it out and taking a good look at it. Find out how it works. If it's battery operated, make sure the battery is charged. Lower and raise the gurney a couple of times to get comfortable with it.

There will be a lot of equipment on a fully stocked gurney. Depending on what crew was on before you, be careful and aware of lazy people not replacing equipment on the gurney. It will always fall on you once you get on scene and realize you are missing equipment! Ask what should be on the gurney at all times. On a call, you don't want to have to run back outside to the ambulance for equipment that you could have taken with you in the first place. Always restock your gurney!

These are some basic tools and equipment that are on most gurneys:

Blankets: People will be cold, especially older patients. You will be going to calls late at night and early in the morning with all types of weather conditions.

Tarps or sheets: disposable sheets are great for covering patients who are dirty, bloody, or have biohazard fluids all over themselves. This will help keep filth from getting on your gurney or you and your partner. On bleeding or heavily soiled patients, make sure you put down extra sheets, chux, or any material that is waterproof. Carry a nice supply of these on all calls. Tarps or sheets will also keep the rain from getting all your equipment wet on rainy days.

Ready Bed or Carry All: this piece of equipment will help you carry out patients who cannot walk or are oversized. It provides a place where patients can transfer onto and be carried by numerous people. It usually has numerous handles for many people to help with the extrication. Remember you will be on many different scenarios and tight work places so be prepared to have this piece of equipment ready at all times.

Restraints: Either leather or soft, restraints are for patients who are a danger to you and your partner. They are also for patients who are a danger to themselves or are combative. Many times you will arrive on scene and find patients who are under the influence, are in a mentally-altered state, or have some type of brain injury. They cannot control themselves or their arm and hand movements. Restraints will be a must. Make sure they are on gurney.

> *"Tips and Tricks for the new EMT"*
> With a combative or altered patient, always make sure the patient is properly restrained before leaving your partner alone in the back of the ambulance.

"TIPS and Tricks for the new EMT"
With a combative or violent patient, fold a sheet in half, place it over the patients midsection and tie the corners to the gurney. It makes a great straitjacket!! If leather restraints are not available, you can use kerlix gauze to tie hands and feet down.

Portable O2 and supplies: Although you will have an Airway bag with O2 and supplies, your gurney should also have an extra oxygen cylinder that you can hook up to the patient once they are on your gurney. Make sure your portable O2 tank is full and that you have extra airway supplies such as Nasal Cannulas, NonRebreathers, or Nebulizer setups.

Pediatric seats: this piece of equipment is small and most of the time can fit onto your gurney. Store below the gurney on the undercarriage or in the compartment space behind the patient. Pediatrics must be securely fastened onto your gurney.

"Tips and Tricks for the new EMT"
By removing the reservoir from a NRM you can put a nebulizer treatment and administer it via mask if the patient is

unable to hold it. You can even set up a BVM to administer treatment. Ask your medic to show you how to set this up.

Emesis bags: For patients who need to vomit. This piece of equipment should be accessible right away. You never know when an accident will occur. Be ready. I will go over cleanup in the following chapters but you get what I'm saying. Keep a knitting hoop with a biohazard bag on the gurney. This will hold a lot of liquids.

"Tips and Tricks for the new EMT"
If the patient is vomiting and there is nothing you can do about it, hold the patient's head to the side of the rig that has the equipment which is easiest to clean. If they are on the gurney and you are pushing them to the ambulance, do the same. Hold the patient's head and aim for the ground. You can also aim for bystanders that would not clear the scene!! Especially with projectile vomiting!!

"Tips and Tricks for the new EMT"
To create a homemade bib for those vomiting patients, cut a hole about the size of your patient's head in one side of

a large trash bag (close to the top). Place over the head of the patient so the bag hangs from the patient's neck in front of the patient. This will create a support hoop for your patient to vomit in!!

Spit sock: Spit socks are for our uncooperative patients who, you guessed it, like to spit at people. Yes you will be spit on. Welcome to EMS!! This piece of equipment can be taped down to the gurney and ready in a split second.

Seat belts: make sure your gurney has all required and county certified belts and harnesses. All patients must be secured onto the gurney in a safe manner.

IV poles: to hold up IV bags that are attached to patients. Make sure it works properly.

{FAMILIARIZE YOURSELF WITH THE MECHANICS OF YOUR GURNEY}

Floor mounts and handles: Get familiar with where they are in the back of the ambulance. These are what lock the gurney into place once you place it into the ambulance. Practice moving the gurney in and out of the ambulance a couple of times to get comfortable with it.

Brakes: Find out where they are on the gurney and make sure they work. This will hold the gurney in place once you are on scene. It will keep the gurney from rolling away and hold the patient steady when getting onto the gurney. Never trust or rely on the brakes and always keep a hand on the gurney!

Head of stretcher: make sure this part of the gurney goes up and down to allow patients to either sit up or lie down. Most gurneys will color code moving parts as well as pinch points. Locate and get familiar with them.

Foot of stretcher: make sure this part of gurney goes up and down. This is mostly used for shock patients whose legs need to be elevated.

Collapsible part of gurney: this will make the gurney shorter for use in tight places such as elevators. Find the collapsible lever or button, which is usually located at the head of the gurney.

You will use and maneuver the gurney into every place and spot imaginable. When steering the gurney, watch for curbs. Hitting one of these will stop the gurney immediately and the person pushing will get a gurney to the mouth or gut. Remember whoever is in the front is steering and whoever is in the back is pushing. The person pushing should always help when going up curbs or bumpy areas by pushing down on the head of the gurney. This will help the person steering when trying to pick up a heavy gurney over a large curb. Be aware that gurneys do tip over so be careful. Try to stay away from rough terrain and bumpy areas. Always secure the patient properly onto the gurney.

WORDS FROM THE WISE; PROVERBS FROM TODAY'S PARAMEDICS

"Be humble. Check your ego. You don't know it all. There is too much knowledge for you to master even after decades of experience. When you are with someone senior to you, ask questions more than offer solutions. Keep your ears open and hear the lessons that have kept patients and other providers alive. Fight the temptation as a new person to "prove" yourself.

Always learn. Never stop learning. I would remind you to look out for each other. This is such a difficult job emotionally and psychologically. Those of us who have been around EMS for 20-plus years have known more than a few people who have committed suicide. There is never an ounce of shame in saying, 'You know, today was a little much for me to handle and I need to talk with a peer-counselor or a mental health professional."

– Tim Kaye (EMT / Paramedic) 16 years experience.

"I would say on the first day just keep it simple. Show up early to familiarize yourself with the apparatus and where things are. As far as rig, know how to use the siren, lights

& gurney. When it comes to knowing where things are, you don't have to necessarily memorize where everything is but do a thorough checkout of your ambulance so you don't look completely lost when someone asks you to get something. Be open to everyone and everything that comes your way, allowing yourself to embrace different possibilities, opportunities, people, views, suggestions, and interests. You need to be unprejudiced, without stubbornness, and be flexible at all times. It's about understanding someone's point of view, even when you disagree or don't like the person."

– **Mike Fields (Fire Fighter / Paramedic) 15 years experience.**

"The most important skill necessary to the success of a new EMT on any EMS crew is communication, both verbal and non-verbal. There will be times you will make mistakes. It happens to everyone. Owning up to the mistakes and telling the truth may result in discipline, but remember the goal of discipline is to correct behavior. I have seen far too many employees lose their jobs/livelihood because of lies. The saddest thing is that the infractions committed wouldn't have resulted in the same outcome had the employee not lied. Your character and reputation will follow you throughout your career. Make it one of honor, trust, and mutual respect."

– Herb Lee (Fire Fighter / Paramedic) 12 years experience.

"I remember my first day as an EMT on the ambulance and remember feeling nervous and not quite knowing what to expect. Many of the skills you learned in EMT school will be helpful, however there is so much more you will learn. Be humble. We are given the unfortunate opportunity to see people at their worst: drunk, bloody, or just alone and at death's door. Bedside manner is huge and is a real skill. You can't fake caring about someone. They don't know that you're getting held over, that you haven't eaten a real meal all day, or that you haven't slept for three days. And if someone is spitting on you, calling you names, etc, don't take it personal. Just deal with it calmly and professionally. Place them in restraints and have an easy ride to the ER. Easy money. This can be a tough job that can drag you down with the weight of dead children and mean drunks. Relax, keep your head up and your eyes and ears open. Be kind to your patients and hopefully one day when you are old and sick you will be paid in good karma."

– **Chris Fraser (Fire Fighter / Paramedic)
19 years experience.**

DRIVING

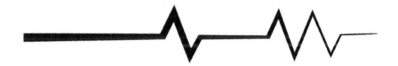

As an EMT, driving will be one of your primary jobs. Let's face it—if you're working 911, the majority of calls will need ALS intervention, which leaves you driving. On scene you will be able to use your EMT skills, but once your patient is stabilized and ready to be loaded, your job is to get your partner and patient to the hospital in a safe and timely manner. You can go from zero to 100 in a matter of seconds. Never let your guard down and get too comfortable. Stay alert and always be ready for action.

"Tips and Tricks for the new EMT"
Get plenty of rest before your shift. Nobody likes a grumpy person. Remember you will have to sit with somebody for 12

hours and sometimes longer than that. Falling asleep behind the wheel is very dangerous. It is your job and responsibility to get rest.

Know the area before you get hired. Drive around your county and learn the highways and how to get to the hospitals. Most companies will have GPS, but do not rely on machines that may fail. There is nothing better than EMT's who know where they are going. Your medic can't be treating a critical patient and directing you to the hospital at the same time. Once you start driving, start to look for landmarks in your area such as mountains and tall buildings to get your bearings when trying to get to hospitals. The pressure to get your checklist completed will overwhelm you when trying to get to the hospital with a critical patient, so knowing where you are going is a great help. People who don't know the area and where they are going are the ones who have the toughest time in EMS. And when I say checklist, I mean that driving is only part of your job in treatment of your patient. You will also be doing the following:

1. Ring downs (pre-hospital reports): this involves a brief summary of what you are bringing to the hospital. Including the sta-

tus of patient, changes, interventions, vital signs, and the ETA (Estimated Time of Arrival).

2. Operating lights and sirens while going through red lights and oncoming traffic.

3. Talking with dispatch and advising them about your status.

4. Talking to your partner about upcoming bumps in the road, patient status, and ETA to hospital. Always give your partner a heads up when you are getting close to the hospital. This will allow them time to complete their patient care.

5. Navigating. You have to know where you are going in a critical situation. It is very important to also know what type of patients can go where. For example, in my county there is only one hospital for burn patients, and there are certain hospitals that can't take stroke or cardiac patients.

"Tips and Tricks for the new EMT"
Be nice to your dispatch. They control your day. Do you want to have a normal workday or be run to the ground with calls and move ups??

Do you know how to use a map book? You need to. Believe me, on that stressful, critical call, the GPS will malfunction and you will need to have a map book available. Again this is important to do before your first day of training. Don't depend on technology—it will fail you.

MAPPING YOUR PARTNER

There will be times when you are not driving and you will probably be doing paperwork in the passenger seat. As you are doing your paperwork you may get a call. This will be your time to effectively map your partner to the call you are dispatched to. Whether you have a computer with GPS or still using a map book you will need to lead them to your destination. First, find where your location and which direction you need to go. Good communication is a must here. Point them in the way they should go and be their eyes as they are driving with their lights and sirens on. Through every intersection you must clear them lane by lane, meaning you are looking out for any cars coming in your direction that are not stopping. You will also need to give them warning streets as they are approaching the destination.

PARKING

When arriving on scene you are responsible for parking the vehicle. Remember to put the vehicle in park before stepping onto the hectic scene!!! Breathe and pay attention. Remember to lock the ambulance at all times. You must be aware that you may have to leave in a hurry. You never want to trap yourself in an area. On calls where there will be a lot of personnel such as fire, police, and possibly your supervisors, you want to make sure you can get out in a hurry. You also want to be safe because most of the vehicle accidents you are called to will be on the freeway or at busy intersections. Think of where you will be loading up your patient and the possibility of getting hit by a car. Park at the tail end of the fire truck. That's usually where your patient's house is. Also if you are on a dead end street or court, never park behind fire trucks. They may get another call like a fire and need to leave quickly. If you are still on scene with the patient you will not be able to move the ambulance until you have loaded them up. Always park in front or to the side of fire trucks so that they can back up. Don't box them in. Teamwork always!!

"Tips and Tricks for the new EMT"
Always back your ambulance with a backer. This means having somebody stand in the rear of the vehicle and direct you into the parking spot. If you are at a hospital and see another ambulance

coming in, back them into the parking space. Be pro-active.

POSTING

In EMS you will sometimes have down time or time when you are not running calls. Dispatch will have you posted or stationary in a certain area. Some of you will have a quarters, house, or fire station where you may be able to sit down and warm up some food. For those of you who will not have these benefits, you will be posted on a street corner. This means you will be sitting in your ambulance during your shift. The key thing here is safety. Don't place yourself in a dark area or an area with potential high crime rates... find a safe place.

SPEEDING

On a critical call, it is your responsibility to get to the hospital in a safe and timely manner. One of the most important things medics like to see is an EMT who is safe. Don't speed!!! Let me say that again: Don't Speed!!! You and your partner want to get home that night. It is all about safety. You will get to the hospital. Don't speed there. Get good at easing into your brakes and easing into your acceleration.

YOUR PATIENT IS LOADED, NOW WHAT?

Once your patient is loaded, you are now ready to get to the hospital. You must determine in your mind (most of this decision making is on scene) what kind of call this is—critical (immediate or code 3) or non critical (non immediate or code 2) . If you don't know or aren't sure then ask your partner. Pay attention on scene!!

After you load the patient into the back of the ambulance and jump into the front seat, then ask your partner if he or she is ready. But before you do that, ask yourself, "Are you ready?" Do you know where you are? Do you know how to get out of the area? Do you know where the closest hospital is and how to get there? Find out all this information first!! Don't just start driving. Getting lost will only make things worse. I understand if this is a critical patient you might feel the need to hurry, but you must know where you're going first. If your partner is shouting at you to go, let him or her know you are mapping yourself. Believe me your partner will appreciate that more than you just driving and getting lost. I've had so many trainees just get in the ambulance, turn on the lights and sirens, and start driving. They don't even know which way to go! Yes the adrenaline will be pumping, but take a deep breath, relax, and map yourself before you start driving.

If all else fails and you're completely lost then you might have to humble yourself and ask your partner to help you. That's why it is so important as you are driving to a call, memorize how you are getting there and how you are going to get out! Start thinking what hospital is closest as you are driving to a call. After mapping yourself to the hospital there will be many other things you will have to do. Get ready to multitask.

"Tips and Tricks for the new EMT"
Learn your counties chart of ten codes. Your communication center or dispatch may use a variety of these over the radio. Ten codes are used to communicate efficiently. (Ex.; 10-4 means that you acknowledge the message or that the message was received.)Each county and agency may differ.

THE PRE-REPORT

One of the many things you will have to do on a call is to give the hospital a pre-report. This means a report on what complaint or condition the patient you're bringing to the hospital is in. It is very important on scene that you pay close attention to what is going on and that you listen to pertinent information. Sometimes you will even do a ring down, or pre-hospital report, on scene. Critical patients, or calls that are less than five minutes away from the hospital, may require this.

As you prepare to give the hospital a report, make sure you have proper training on how to use the radio and what channels you need to be on in order to talk to the hospital. Some counties will require you to call on the phone. It is very important you have all phone numbers to hospitals stored on your company or personal phone. Make sure you have all the information to give the hospital before you call or ring down. I mentioned two-inch tape onto the pant leg might look funny but will save you in a stressful moment. Writing on gloves is not the best alternative. You will eventually throw them away, along with all the information that was on them. This just happens, trust me. This is a great example of how important it is to keep the cab of the ambulance super clean. The cab is where you and your partner will spend most of the day. The last thing you want to do is jump up front and start driving with dirty gloves contaminating the steering wheel, radio, and everything else in your office.

As you prepare to give the hospital a pre-report, always make sure you are on the same page as your partner regarding the condition of the patient. You and your partner may have a different interpretation of what the chief complaint is so double check with your partner if you are not sure. It is also good to communicate if there are any updates on your patients (i.e., now they are getting CPR, they have a pulse, there's a change in vital signs, etc.). Once you have your info then you can radio or call the hospital. Be clear with the report and always give an ETA (estimated time of arrival).

GETTING TO THE HOSPITAL

Once your report is done, now you can start to drive. You don't have to speed. Your priority is to get your partner, the patient, and yourself to the hospital safely. You are responsible for many lives on a call. Most of the time you will have to take extra personnel, such as extra medics or firefighters. Sometimes you will even have family members of the patient with you.

> *"Tips and Tricks for the new EMT"*
> **When driving always have an eye on your partner in the back of the ambulance. A good EMT can watch his medic in the back with a patient, drive code 3, talk to dispatch, map themselves, and ring down the hospital...all while comforting the patient's family member in the passenger seat!**

Another priority is to make sure your partner can get his or her job done efficiently and smoothly in the back. If you're driving like a maniac, all you will be doing is throwing your partner around. Again, medics hate crazy and out-of-control drivers, and most medics will not be using seat belts. Pay attention to your rear view mirror. It's not only there to look at cars behind you but also to keep an eye out for your partner. Pay attention to what is going on back there. Is your driving stopping your partner from doing effective CPR, intubations, or starting IV's? Most medics will yell out when they are starting an IV or doing a procedure that requires a steady hand or smooth driving. Pay attention because you may have to slow down or stop. With combative and uncooperative patients, always be looking in the back. Your partner may need you to stop and jump in back to help. You will get better as time goes on.

> *"Tips and Tricks for the new EMT"*
> *If a backboard is handy restrain all combative patients to it and not to the gurney. That way when you get to the hospital, all you have to do is lift them over and place them on the hospital bed. No fighting, no problem!*

Once your partner is ready to go, ask if you are going to the hospital with lights and sirens or not, meaning is it a critical call or is the patient stable? You should already know but being new you will need some time to identify sick versus really sick. If you don't know the severity of the call it's important to communicate with your partner on how you will be getting to the hospital. Never be afraid to ask if you don't know. If you don't think you have the right information, just ask. There is nothing worse than somebody who pretends to know what they are doing. You will be found out, usually on a critical and stressful call. Don't be ashamed to ask your partner—you are learning, and he or she will understand you are new and need a little help. Your partner will appreciate your honesty and eagerness to learn, rather than if you pretend to know and then mess up vital information.

Now that you are ready to go to the hospital, you may be driving code 3 (lights and sirens)—if so, turn them on! Once you turn on Code 3 lights and sirens, some vehicles will follow the proper procedures of pulling over so you can maneuver through and some will not. Be patient. Your stress and anger levels can get the best of you here with drivers not knowing the proper laws and rules when being approached by an ambulance. Your sirens will give them the hint and most ambulances will have an intercom. Stay professional, don't get angry, and stay calm. Be careful of cars that will pull out in front of you or to the wrong side of the road. You will have to maneuver through with caution.

Once in a while you will have to brake hard so be in constant communication with your partners and let them know when there will be a hard stop! You will also have to watch out for bumps and train tracks on the road. Going over these will require you to yell out to your partner "TRACKS" or "BUMP." Again you must be watching in back. You don't want to hit a bump as your partner is starting an IV or doing some type of important ALS intervention. This will alert your partners that they must brace themselves. In critical situations, your hard stops and bumps could

prevent a successful IV and meds given to your patient. Be careful. Driving with lights and sirens doesn't mean you drive faster. It will allow you to move cars out of the way and go through red lights but be careful. When going through red lights, make sure you make a full stop. Look both ways and clear each lane one by one. Before proceeding into intersections, use the proper sirens, wailers, and yelps to alert all drivers that you are coming through. Remember you are requesting they move out of the way. It doesn't mean they will do it. I will not go further into driving. The company that hires you will have some sort of driving program that you must go through to prove you know what you are doing and are safe.

FAMILY MEMBERS

Other things to consider when going to the hospital are family members that want to ride with you. Initially, out of the kindness of your heart and compassion to help them, you are going to want to let family members ride with you to the hospital. Most of the time it's okay. Just make sure you and your partner both agree. Sometimes we don't let family members ride with us because of the emotions they feel when their loved one is sick or clinging on to life. Stress levels and anxiety are at an all-time high. When people get emotional they sometimes lose control and this will affect your job and the care a patient receives.

Family members who are over the top, hysterical, freaking out, or drunk are too dangerous to come with you. Most family members who are like this will interfere with your patient care and make the situation worse. I've had family members yelling and screaming at us to do something about their family members. They don't understand what we are doing, which can interfere with our patient care. They yell and freak out about the route we are taking to the hospital. They complain we are driving too slow and demand that we drive faster. They yell at your partners in the back about how to do their jobs. They yell out to their loved ones in distress. We have compassion and understand the emotions but these people are interfering with our patient care and should not be in the ambulance. Kindly ask that they take their personal cars to the hospital. If you have time, give or draw out directions to the hospital for them. You can also ask other EMS personnel to give them directions.

Once you are able to convince family members to drive themselves to the hospital, you will have another problem—family members following too closely. Usually when you are driving with lights and sirens on, you will have a critical patient on board. You will be going through red lights and getting to the hospital as fast as you can in a safe manner. This will be the time that family member wants to follow you through every red light. They will tailgate you and you'll feel like they are on top of your bumper. This is unsafe for everybody. Although you will not be able to stop them, you can politely ask them before you go to the hospital not to follow you. You can even ask them to go before you. At minimum, let them know you will be driving with lights and sirens on and that you will be traveling quickly and through red lights. Let them know the dangers of following you. Remind them to obey the traffic laws.

Now that you have taken care of that, continue on with your patient care. On some calls you will be taking extra personnel or healthcare workers to help your partner in the back. Before leaving, make sure your partner has all the necessary hands he or she needs to take care of the patient. Make sure you have all the pertinent information for the patient that your partner and hospital will need. Sometimes your partners will be so busy stabilizing the patient that you will be their saving grace. It's very important you have the patient's information such as medical history, meds, ID, and insurance cards.

> ## "Tips and Tricks for the new EMT"
> When flying out a patient on a helicopter make sure you know where the Landing Zone is. These are usually hectic and nerve-wrecking calls. Ask the fire department to take you there or make sure you have directions. You don't want to get lost on calls like these.

Before you leave, always double check and make sure your equipment doesn't get left on scene. Do another inspection of the area if possible. On critical calls, it will be a "load and go" so forgetting equipment at the scene is possible. As the patient is loaded up, it is your job before you start driving away to make sure that all equipment is in the rig and all info is collected for the hospital. Remember your partner's mind is on assessing the patient. In a car accident, for example, make sure you get a good look at the car and how much damage has occurred. This will help your medic at the hospital when giving a turnover report. Your partner may have missed something that you didn't. Many times you will be the medic's eyes and ears! Even taking pictures of the wreck will help the trauma doctor's assessment. Just remember to not take pictures of patients due to HIPPA, which sets rules about who can look at and receive patients' health information. Once the patient is loaded up, always let your partner know you are going to make last minute observations of the wreck. Airbag deployment, starring of windshield, steering wheel deformity—all the stuff you should have learned in EMT school. All these notes will help your partner with his or her assessment.

"Tips and Tricks for the new EMT"
Always walk on scene with a smile. Your first impression sets the atmosphere for this call. Come in with a great attitude and again smile... smiles go a long way in EMS.

WORDS FROM THE WISE; PROVERBS FROM TODAY'S PARAMEDICS

"Do not tell your medic how you would do things or try to prove how much you know. As a new EMT, being very attentive and able to follow instructions is key. I worked with a newer EMT the other day and had to repeat myself several times and ended up doing things myself because he was too slow. Don't be afraid to ask if you don't know something. Asking a partner questions about something you don't know is much better that not asking and risking making big mistakes."
– John Sagli (Fire Fighter / EMT Paramedic) 10 years experience.

"I remind EMT's that I first work with that despite what some medics might think, I believe you as the EMT has the more important role because I can only kill one of us (the patient), you can kill us all. I think the most important thing I usually say to new EMT partners is, I'm pretty easy. Don't worry about hanging me an IV bag or tossing me around back here; I'm not fra-gee-le. And however you want to get to the call or transport to the hospital is fine with me. Take a deep breath and remember: this ain't rocket science! You know why? Because we don't get paid like rocket scientists'."

– Jeff Lingao (EMT / Paramedic) 14 years experience.

"I remember my first shift as an EMT, so many years ago, like it was yesterday. I remember how nervous I was to be finally on my own, not wanting to make any mistakes. Medics are a sensitive type and if anything is out of their normal, it adds stress and the first person that is going to be blamed is the new EMT. Every shift, regardless of who I was working with, I went and grabbed all that I could to get the ambulance RFA. I would find out how he/she liked the ambulance to be set up. Where do they want the ECG patches, where do they want IV set ups, do they prefer a pre-spike bag or not? Do they use locks instead of hanging a bag on every patient? Do they like to have tape pre-cut to size? The first day is going to be very thrilling and you're not going to be any good the first time out. Take a deep breath and remember, we only look like we know what we're doing because we've made more mistakes than you."

– Shawn Ellis (EMT / Paramedic) 15 years experience.

"Take a deep breath. Not every call is a major trauma or code. When you go on scene also be looking at exit plans. The way you came in may not be the best way out. I.e., is the backyard through the slider easier than the stairs you had to lift the gurney up? Your partner will appreciate having that figured out already. If you have ANY doubt about route to hospital, ask. Don't get us lost. It's a fun, cool job. It's okay to be excited and love it but always be professional. Remember, if you didn't make it worse, learn from it and move forward."

– Jaci Viskochil (EMT / Paramedic) 18 years experience.

"I feel that being on the same page as your partner is one of the most important traits. It can take normally a few shifts if not months to figure your partner out. One thing you can do is be prepared. Carry that pair of shears, wear that radio and pager. Last thing anyone wants to do is look dumb or unprepared. So if you stay ready you won't have to get ready. We know you're new and most of us have worked with plenty of new people. Don't be afraid to make some decisions. Learn your area. If you're unsure of where you are and you have some time open a map book. Also regardless of what Albert says you do have to abide by most of the DMV handbook. So don't drive like a total jackass FNG."

— **Loren Sakai (EMT / Paramedic) 12 years experience.**

"Congratulations! You have begun to have an amazing career. The really exciting calls are amazing, exhilarating, and we all live off the rush of adrenaline that we feel when running calls. This you will soon experience and understand. However, please do not forget the most mundane, boring routine call. The one where someone's grandmother hurt her hip again, or suffered a fall. These are equally important. Remember you have no understanding of their life so leave your judgement at the door. Even though we perceive "their emergency" to be routine, it might be life altering to them. Do not minimize their feelings and always remember that that everyone is someone to somebody. Even the stinky intoxicated person lying on the ground. The things you see and will endure will ultimately shape who you are as a person. Remember you will make mistakes—they are opportunities to grow and learn. Be humble, possess integrity, and ask questions, always!"

— **Sue Stapleton (EMT / Paramedic) 17 years experience.**

"Most important thing: Be humble and willing to learn. You don't know as much as you think you do. If you don't know something, it's OK, please say so early! Words of advice: remember this excitement level and feeling right now! Harness it and never forget you are here to help people....be grateful and willing to help them. Always be teachable and willing to learn. Stay humble and have fun."
– **Captain Michael Lacy (Fire Fighter / Paramedic) 19 years experience.**

"I would like EMT's to be relaxed and confident in their skills. The individual does not need any additional stress or pressure from me. The more calls the individual runs, the more experience the individual will get in EMS. The less stressful of an environment I can create for the new EMT, the better they will perform under high pressure situations. This also fosters a good working relationship between the two of us."
– **Issac Quevedo (EMT / Paramedic) 18 years experience.**

"I guess I would say be honest about your skills and assume nothing. Nobody expects you to know everything the first day, but you gotta be honest about where you are still learning. For example, don't drive around lost. Ask for help from your partner, fire, dispatch, etc.. Don't assume other people know what is going on. If something seems unclear or wrong about a patient or situation, speak up! When I used to train new hires as an FTO, my big push was not to see if you could do everything but rather to see if you could communicate and use your resources correctly. Work your way through the unknown in a safe, efficient manner."

– Ryan Dean (Flight Nurse / EMT) 15 years experience.

"My number one thing is everyone gets a pillow and a blanket. 95% of this job is hand holding. Show compassion to everyone. The frequent flyer/drunk is still going to call 911 no matter how you treat them. Make everyone comfortable. Wear your uniform and have a presentable gurney. Straps buckled and tucked under. Sloppy pants inside and unzipped boots are unacceptable. No untucked or faded T-shirts. Know your district and every way to every hospital. You are not the first person to be in this position. Speak up if something critical is going to happen but unless you know exactly what your medic is thinking, keep quiet and ask " WHY" after the call. Don't be a know-it-all. Have fun. This really is a job that you make what you will of it. Remember you signed up for this. That happy-go-lucky attitude needs to continue for your career."

– Cardiff Schmitz (Fire Fighter / Paramedic) 12 years experience

ON SCENE

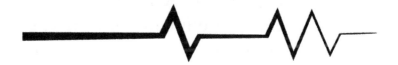

"Tips and Tricks for the new EMT"
A good EMT knows the Paramedics every move. They are pretty much a ninja!

Before we step on the scene of a call, I have to address something with us EMT's. Paramedics have the highest level of authority and care when you are on the scene of a call. It is their patient and they will do the initial assessment. I know some of you EMT's are anxious to get in there and take care of the patient. That's awesome. But hopefully after this chapter you will see how important your role on scene really is. Let the pride and ego go and accept the fact that you are the paramedic's assistant. If you want to run the scene, then go to paramedic school. And if some of you have been to paramedic school, you probably are still not accredited to run calls. I hate to put it like that but some EMT's cause more problems for their partners by interfering and getting in the way of the initial assessment. As it is, some scenes are chaotic, so help your partner by assisting them with what they need. By the end of the chapter, I hope to educate you on your role so much that you will look at your role in a whole new light.

On the scene of a call there will be someone attending to the patient and one assisting. The combination of the EMS providers will differ all around the world. Most common and for the purpose of this book it will be the

Paramedic and EMT-B on an ambulance. Other counties will be staffed with one AEMT or EMT-I and one EMT-B or EMR. If the ambulance is staffed with 2 EMT'S-B's then whoever is attending to the patient will have patient care and the other will assist.

Have your partners back and help them!! The most important part to being an EMT is knowing your role on scene. Let me give you a sneak peek of your role on scene during a call in case you think an EMT's job is not important:

1. Driving code 3 with lights and sirens and mapping to the call (hopefully you have GPS).

2. Monitoring the radio for dispatch instructions and hitting proper buttons to notify them of your status and time stamps.

3. Securing the ambulance and making sure it is locked at all times.

4. Getting the gurney out and placing it as close to the patient as possible.

5. BLS skills and initial encounter with the patient (taking vital signs, administering first aid, controlling bleeding, hooking up to EKG monitor, setting your partner up with proper tools to administer meds, etc). Learn how to set up your patient on a monitor. Learn how to use the automated BP cuff, O2 sensor, and capnography. Learn where leads go on a patient when using an EKG monitor and also know how to apply 12 lead patches for a patient.

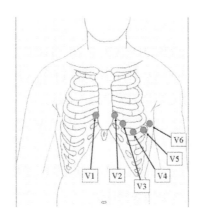

"Tips and Tricks for the new EMT"
When applying the EKG patches, remember "Clouds over the grass" (white over green) and "Smoke over fire" (black over red)

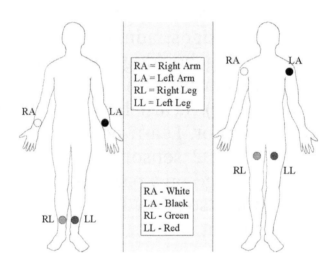

RA = Right Arm
LA = Left Arm
RL = Right Leg
LL = Left Leg

RA - White
LA - Black
RL - Green
LL - Red

6. If the first responder is there first, ask them how you can assist and getting in there to help until they transfer care to you.

7. Getting info (meds, history, allergies, ID, insurance cards, etc.).

8. Getting the patient to the gurney. Assisting with walking or carrying.

9. Getting equipment off scene and back in the ambulance.

10. Loading the patient into the ambulance and continuing to help your partner stabilize the patient in the back of the ambulance. This is done before you drive off.

11. Advising dispatch of status and pushing proper buttons for time stamp.

12. Calling or ringing down hospital with pre-hospital report.

13. Driving code 3 with lights and sirens and mapping yourself to hospital.

14. Unloading patient.

> *"Tips and Tricks for the new EMT"*
> *If you think you might need a cop, you probably already should have called for one. If you think a patient needs to be restrained, restrain them!*

This is just a few of your roles on scene!!! If you're worried about not being involved in the call, think again.

Your role is very important.

> *"Tips and Tricks for the new EMT"*
> *Whenever you get a chance, use the restroom. You do not want to be on a call*

when the greasy lunch starts to churn in your stomach!

So you've arrived to the area of your call. As you drive to the scene of your call, you must be thinking of a number of things before you get off your ambulance. Is the scene safe?

Yes, the stuff you learned in EMT school is for real. You will encounter every type of scene imaginable. Assaults, violent crimes, and combative patients are some situations you will face. Remember, you and your partner's safety is the top priority. Road hazards, downed telephone wires, smoke, fires, and leakage from hazardous materials are all real dangers you will approach. You have to make sure your scene is safe before getting off of your ambulance. Police or fire will usually clear the scene and deem it safe to come in. Wait for these orders.

"Tips and Tricks for the new EMT"
If you hear these words...
CODE BROWN = potential or possibly has diarrhea or defecated
CODE YELLOW = potential or possibly has urinated
VOMIT = they are about to vomit. Never stand in front of somebody about to throw up!

BEWARE AND TAKE PRECAUTIONS ASAP

Once the scene is safe you can now assess the situation. When receiving a call, you will usually have a little info. Bring suspected equipment so you don't have to come all the way back to your ambulance when making initial contact. Upon making contact with the patient you have to be asking yourself if this person is sick or stable. Will we be leaving quickly or stabilizing the patient on scene? Yes, the famous "Stay and play, or load and go?" You will always have to be thinking, "How are we going to get this patient out of here?" Just keep that in mind as you approach your patient. You will assist your partner in treating the patient but you have a lot of other responsibilities you need to be thinking about as well. Let's go through them:

1. You will have to perform most BLS skills for your partner. This means when you approach the patient, get in there and perform the necessary treatment. You should know how to attach the patient to an EKG monitor and learn how to set up a 12 lead EKG for your partner. You should be familiar with setting up to get blood sugar, temperature, albuterol treatment, and CPAP. Even though you can't perform ALS interventions you should know how to set up for every single one.

Ask your medic to show you how. Learning the medications and how to set them up for administration are also very important. Remember your scope of practice. Most counties don't allow certain things to be done by an EMT so know your county's policies and protocols. But by setting up your partners with their tools, they will be more efficient in their patient care. Don't forget, most people on scene of a call will know you are new. They will know if you know what you are doing. Don't fake it...they will see right through you. It's OK. They want to help you but only if you're humble and transparent enough to receive it.

"*Tips and Tricks for the new EMT*"
Learn how to point and say "PAIN" in several different languages
Spanish : Dolor
Chinese : tongs tong
Arabic : alam
Hindi : dard
Portuguese : dor
Russian : bol
Japanese : Itami
Vietnamese : dau don

2. Once the patient is stabilized or help arrives for your partner (fire, police, or another EMS agency), you have to be thinking how to get the

patient to the gurney and into the ambulance. You will always want to bring the gurney as close to the patient as possible. Be thinking about the positioning of the gurney. Will they bring the patient out head first or feet first? When carrying a patient down flights of stairs and out of the house, this will help tremendously. Think, do I have seat belts ready, a pediatric seat ready, restraints for combative patients? Do I have enough sheets and soak proof material for heavy bleeding patients? Believe me, getting the gurney ready will help your call and cleanup run smoothly.

3. As you are on scene of your call, you have to be thinking what hospital is most appropriate for this patient and which hospital is closest. Do we fly them out on an aircraft or do we drive them? It is very important to know all your trauma centers, burn centers, psych facilities, etc. This will really impress your FTO on your training time. Most importantly you should know how to get to all your county's hospitals!

4. Do we have all pertinent information such as meds, history, and allergies? And are we forgetting any important info such as DNR paperwork, ID, or insurance cards?

5. At some point, you will have a scene where the patient cannot walk. As these patients are being stabilized you have to start thinking, "Will we carry them out? How are we going to carry them

out? What type of equipment will I need to carry them out?" Determining the weight of the patient is also a big factor. It will determine how many people you need to help with lifting the patient and what type of equipment you will need to get him or her out. If you need to leave to get the necessary equipment, communicate with your partner first and let him or her know. It is up to you to prepare to get the patient out.

> _**"Tips and Tricks for the new EMT"**_
> **ABC'S OF EMS = Ambulate Before Carry. We try and use our backs as less as possible. If the patient can walk with assistance then let them walk.**

6. Recognize the difficulty you will have maneuvering the gurney to the patient. Many times you will have to maneuver your gurney through the obvious: doors, ramps, stairs, grass, dirt, water, mud, snow, and wind. You will find that some gurneys cannot be carried up flights of stairs (especially motorized gurneys). You will also find that most gurneys don't fit down small hallways and some elevators will not fit a gurney into it. You will have to carry out patients to the gurney so always be thinking, "How can I get this gurney closest to the patient?" Be aware of your surroundings and weather conditions. Always have

equipment on your gurney such as carry all stretchers or transfer flats, extra blankets, and sheets.

"Tips and Tricks for the new EMT"
Always make sure your gurney looks presentable when stepping on the scene. This means clean sheet and seat belts buckled. Disposable pillow in place with disposable blankets and sheets folded nicely somewhere on gurney. Make a good impression the minute you get on scene.

Once your gurney is in the right position, with seatbelts unattached and handrails down, go back and assist with the extrication of the patient. If the patient is coming downstairs it is very important that there is enough help carrying the patient. You will hear it over and over again that in EMS, the No. 1 injury is back injuries. You must be careful when carrying patients, especially downstairs. The person or persons carrying the patient's head will have the heaviest side. Assist with that. Also keep in mind that people at the bottom cannot see where they are going when carrying people down the stairs. You will have to be their guide down the stairs, constantly in communication. Even placing your hand behind their backs and giving them audible directions is greatly appreciated. Constant stretching and working out before a shift will help you tremendously with this part of your job. Take care of your back!!

Once patients are on the gurney, make sure they are secured with the proper seat belts. Place the patient on a monitor, give them O2, and adjust the gurney according to the treatment (shock position, for example). Maneuvering the gurney with a patient on it can be very tricky. That is why it is your job to determine the best path for extricating patients and loading them onto the ambulance. Also, constant communication with your partner is important. One of you will be steering and the other will be pushing. Be careful with curbs, uneven asphalt, and rocks. The gurney with a patient on it will be top-heavy, so the possibility of the patient falling over is great. Sometimes you will still be performing ALS interventions while the patient is on gurney, such as controlling bleeding, administering CPR, or giving medications. Load the patient into the back of the ambulance and hop in the back with your partner.

"Tips and Tricks for the new EMT"
For our fake unconscious patients who will not cooperate with our assessments,

a good ol' sternal rub or pen to the bottom of the foot will usually do the trick. Eyelashes are very ticklish and you will usually get a response from this. Lube up the ol' NPA and perform your BLS skill with a smile. An arm drop across their face will usually cause their heads to move right before it hits them.

Continue stabilizing and treating the patient with your partner. On every call, you and your medic will have to decide who will care for the patient. Let's keep this simple and to the point. If it's an ALS complaint then the medic should tech it. If it's BLS you should not even have to be asked if you want to tech the call. You should already be in the back of the ambulance with patient. Remember working ALS, will obviously have your medic attending most of the calls. It is important to try to give him or her a break once in awhile. Don't just be a taxi driver, be an EMT.

"Tips and Tricks for the new EMT"
If you need to write down information on patient and you don't have a notepad, write on towels, chux, or 4x4's. You can even write on the disposable gurney sheets that the patient is sitting or laying on.

Once your medic is readyto go, make one more tour of the area where you treated the patient. It is so important you don't leave equipment on scene. Also try to clean up the area, and most importantly, make sure all needles are secure and stored away in containers for sharp objects. Sometimes on hectic calls, the medics will forget to put away or store needles in the proper containers. You don't want anybody to get poked with a needle.

Now you are ready to go to the hospital. Remember to put your seat belt on and notify dispatch of where you are going. Get ready to call the hospital and give a report of what you are bringing. As I said before, it is very important that you are paying attention the minute you arrive at the scene. Find out what happened and know the story. Listen to what the chief complaint is. Know what procedure and intervention is being performed on the patient. You will be giving the hospital a prehospital report so at minimum you should know the following:

1. Chief Complaint
2. What happened?
3. Vital signs
4. Patient's current condition
5. Care given to patient

6. ETA

Remember your partner will be busy with the patient and should not have to tell you what to say to the hospital.

A couple of other things to consider on scene of calls:

1. Patients who die at the scene should be left in the position in which you gave care. You can clean up material around patients that was used to care for them and then wait until law enforcement arrives. You can cover patients with a sheet or blanket. Family members may want to spend time with the deceased so be sensitive to that.

2. Remain calm on scene and in control of your emotions. Always take deep breaths and control your breathing. Keep the adrenaline down. Remember you are doing your best to take care of the patient and that's all you can do. Rushing and running around on scene will add to the chaos and confusion. Remain calm and be confident you are doing your best.

3. You will be working with many other departments and agencies. This is a team effort. Do your best to get along and work

with each other. The patient is the primary concern of the team on scene.

4. Maintain your composure. You will see everything your school told you about. The horror story calls and traumatic events are all real. You will see children in critical situations and families in distress. Do your best to remain professional.

"Tips and Tricks for the new EMT"
People who get pepper sprayed will require a lot of water. Your ambulance won't have the amount needed to flush the eyes. If possible find a water hose close by in a residential home and spray your patient down. That works much better.

WORDS FROM THE WISE; PROVERBS FROM TODAY'S PARAMEDICS

This line of work has multiple influences contributing to not only the call that you're on but for the entire shift that you are working. Doesn't matter how well you prepare or try to mitigate other influences, stuff is still going to not go right. My advice, take a few deep breaths, acknowledge what's going wrong, attempt to correct it, don't beat yourself up over it to the point where you get distressed. Distressed EMS workers make mistakes and don't manage stress well.

The mindset of your paramedic partner.That blob of human flesh sitting in the passenger's seat next to you is called a paramedic. This poor soul has endured mind numbing education and is ALWAYS under multiple layers of stress. Some medics manage this stress well, some not so well. You have little control over this so just roll with whatever personality type of medic partner you get. Hint: the more helpful you are and the more you actually pay attention to what's going on, the more you will soften up even the saltiest medic partner. Ultimately your medic is held accountable for everything that happens on that ambulance. If the poo hits the fan, it's your medic that gets the phone call first. This applies to everything: patient care/outcome, interagency relations, equipment failure and any kind of complaints.

It's normal to feel a degree of anxiety when you're a new EMT. Here are a couple of things that you can do in the beginning of your career to smooth that bumpy road.

1) Wholeheartedly, strive to be the best 911 EMT in the field. If you have aspirations of becoming a medic someday, you MUST be a great EMT first. So don't skip this step. I've had brand new EMT partners who acted like they were just going through the motions of their job because in their head it was just a brief stepping stone on their way to becoming a "ParaGod." I can tell you with confidence that they were not only poor EMT's but also when they did become medics, they had an extra hard time. The decade that I spent as an EMT, I prided myself with the fact that I was like my medics' surgical nurse. I paid attention to what was happening all the time and was there as an immediate support system to fill in any gaps and complete tasks. I was handing my medics equipment even before they asked for it. Strive to become this way. If you don't know something, ask. If you want to learn something advanced or special, your medic will still be more than willing, but pick an appropriate time.

2) I've always thought that there are usually only two kinds of people who willingly enter the business of 911 EMS: the "Do-Gooder" who wants to help their fellow man and save or help everyone and the "Ricky Rescue" who seeks the excitement and thrill of the occupation. In reality, if you are exclusively one or the other, you're going to be very disappointed and burn out fast in 911 EMS. Speaking as an EMS worker who has over 25 years of experience, it's best to have only a portion of each type, just be yourself, not exclusively a "type." Honestly, the calls that you'll run on a 911 ambulance are for the most part routine, non critical. But there are those calls that will challenge your humanity. If your attitude type is exclusively Ricky Rescue you're not going to be happy and you'll become bored, lazy, and disrespectful and you'll eventually fail because you'll start making mistakes.

If your attitude type is exclusively Do-Gooder, you're not going to be happy either. You'll realize that not everyone can be helped or saved and there is rarely a "thank you" heard. In fact you'll be inundated with hateful/disrespectful comments from people and you'll eventually emotionally implode. Hint: try to keep you as a person separate from the job. Don't become 100% the job.

– **Karen Kleindienst (EMT / Paramedic) 25 years experience.**

UNLOADING THE PATIENT

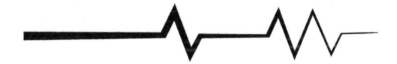

When en route to the hospital, be sure to always record miles. This is how your company will be paid for transport. Always alert your partners when you are approximately 3 to 5 minutes away from the hospital. This will allow them to prepare for the arrival and perform any last minute ALS procedures. Hit all your buttons that will alert dispatch of your status. Remember to turn off all emergency lights. Hospitals like you to turn off your ambulance completely to avoid exhaust flowing into their emergency rooms. Just make sure you advise your partners you are shutting down power. They will likely lose lights in the back of ambulance. When you arrive at the hospital, notify dispatch of your arrival and jump in the back of the ambulance to help your partner.

You will need to assist with any last minute interventions and BLS skills. You will either be bringing equipment with you or disconnecting it from the patient. Don't worry about clean-up just yet. You will have plenty of time to finish that after you unload the patient.

"Tips and Tricks for the new EMT"
Your dispatch will start a timer once you arrive at the hospital. It will usually not be enough time. 3 to 5 minutes before you time out, call for extra time to help with clean up and paperwork.

On a non-critical patient, unloading may not be as fast, compared to unloading a critical patient which will be very fast. You will be managing the gurney, carrying equipment, and performing BLS skills while walking into the hospital. When unloading the patient, make sure all cables and airway equipment are either connected to the patient on gurney or disconnected from the patient and left in the ambulance. Connect airway equipment to the portable o2 (oxygen tank) on the gurney. It is very important that you do not pull out any tubes (endotracheal), Cannulas/NRM, or IV sites connected to the patient.

After your gurney and patient is clear from ambulance connections, start to bring out your gurney with the patient. When unloading make sure the stretcher catches the "hook"when you pull it out of the rig. Your partner should be watching this. Always use two people to take the gurney out. Save your backs! Bring the patient out slowly to ensure proper care, such as CPR or ventilation, can continue. You will have to know the door codes to get into the emergency room. On your FTO time, start taking notes and writing them down. Memorize these door codes. The last thing you want is to be stuck outside with a critical patient.

Your report will have alerted the hospital to where your patient will be going. As you enter the hospital, remember to stay calm and go slow. Rushing or running inside is how IVs get pulled and tubes get displaced from the patient's airway. Understand on a critical call there will be a lot of people waiting for you and watching you come in. Doctors, nurses, police, X-ray techs, and your nosy coworkers will be standing by. Stay calm.

As you enter the room where the patient will be assessed, your partner or whoever is attending to the patient will give the report out loud. Sometimes fire will maintain care and they will give the report. This means you will be transporting firefighters as well. Get the gurney as close to the bed as possible and begin to disconnect all equipment from the patient as hospital workers begin to attach theirs. Do this as quickly as possible and don't forget any of your equipment. Ask patients to cross their arms across their chest and not to grab anything.

> *"Tips and Tricks for the new EMT"*
> *When placing a patient on your gurney who cannot walk, always place something underneath them. You can even use a blanket or bed sheet here. This will help you at the hospital when transferring patients to hospital gurney. You will be able to carry them on this instead of having to pick them up.*

Transfer the patient over to the bed. Usually you will have some type of transfer sheet that the patient is on so all you will need is extra hands to carry patients over. Ask for help from whoever is in the room. Don't worry about who it is. Get help from the doctor if that's who is available. Your back is very important and moving patients is how we get hurt. Get help! Remember to remove seat belts—these tend to be forgotten. Count to three out loud when moving patients over. This will alert everyone to pull or push at the same time. Don't be afraid to take the lead. Once your patient is transferred over, take your gurney and don't forget any equipment. Take your gurney outside and get ready to clean, disinfect, and replace equipment.

CLEAN UP

Most of the time cleanup will be easy and will not require much attention. But once in a while you will get that call that includes blood, urine, feces, or vomit. This will require extra attention. You may need to call your supervisors and get extra time. Regardless of how bad the call is, all gurneys get disinfected afterward, including all equipment like the monitor cables and wires, BP Cuff, etc. For major liquid or fluids on your gurney, you will need to take all equipment off the gurney and give the gurney a major bath. Usually hospitals will have a hose outside the ER bay. They do the same thing with their gurneys. Take all the equipment off and give a rinse down with the hose. Also spray down the gurney mattress. Spray down very thoroughly and especially get into crevices and places where blood and vomit can seep into. This is a very tedious job but you must do it. Your partner will be doing paperwork and most of the time will not be able to help you.

"Tips and Tricks for the new EMT"
Always disinfect the bottom of your boots after horrendous-looking house calls or bloody trauma and fluid-filled

calls. We sometimes forget. You don't want to track these infectious diseases into your stations and into your own homes! Always take your boots off when getting home from a shift!

Some equipment will be badly damaged and will not be reusable, so you will have to get new equipment. Most of the time your supervisors will allow you to be out of service to go back to headquarters and get new equipment. Be sure to know what equipment is needed to stay in service and what you need to be placed out of service. Get a copy or download your county's policy and protocol book. Wipe down all equipment such as EKG monitor leads, BP cuffs, suction equipment, etc. Jump bags where you keep your equipment will have to be cleaned and equipment will have to be replaced that you used on the call. As your gurney and equipment is drying, it's time to get into the back of the ambulance and do a cleanup there. First get all loose garbage out. It will look like a train wreck back there with equipment and wrappers all over the floor and ambulance. Empty packages, bloody wipes, and trauma dressings need to be disposed of properly. All disposable equipment should be replaced after every call in which it is used.

Start to clean up all fluids and liquids off of equipment and the floor. Disinfect everything! In some cases you will even have to mop the floor along with hosing it down. You can only imagine how crazy it can get back there. After disinfecting, start to replace any equipment in airway, trauma, and jump bags. Replace equipment in monitors, suction equipment, and cabinets in the ambulance. Make a list of everything you use during the day. You will have to replace it when you get back to headquarters. There's nothing worse than leaving your relief crew with missing equipment. Use a notepad or stick a piece of cloth tape to the back somewhere. This will insure you don't forget any equipment you have to replace. After every call make sure you write down what you use. At the end of the day you will be able to re-stock your rig efficiently. After everything dries up, start to return all equipment to the gurney and bags. Make sure the gurney has everything back on it. Place the gurney back in the ambulance and get ready for the next call. As your partner is finishing up paperwork and you are through cleaning the gurney and the back of the ambulance, go into the hospital and try to get billing info for your partner.

"Tips and Tricks for the new EMT"
When having to use the restroom at the

hospital, go to the second floor or outside of the E.R. The bathrooms will be twice as clean!!

This will be patient info, billing, and insurance sheets. Usually the registration clerk in ER will help you with this information. The clerk can usually print something out that you can hand to your partner. If not, be sure to write it down and help your partner out. Depending on the call, this may assist your partner with the extra-long report he or she will have to write. You will usually have time after your call to wind down a bit and EAT!!! Use your time wisely. I advise you to pack a meal and snacks. Do not depend on stopping somewhere to get food. It may not happen. It could be so busy that day that you will not be able to stop.

"Tips and Tricks for the new EMT"
If you're lucky enough to get somewhere and order food make sure you get it to go (you will always seem to get a call while eating.) This way you can grab and go!

There is nothing worse than an empty stomach. There is nothing worse than a grumpy EMT. Your time at the hospital will usually be a good time to eat. Once your dispatcher puts you back in service you may not eat for a while after running call, after call, after call, after call........Happy bellies = Happy EMT's and Paramedics = Happy Patients!!

Words from the Wise; Proverbs from Today's Paramedics

"Basically you are coming into a situation, most likely, where the medic has his/her "way" of doing things. This has been developed, through experiences, often through hard lessons learned by the medic through past mistakes. It has become a way to survive the stress, responsibility and unknowns dished out to them daily. Be sensitive to each medic and try to figure out their "way" of doing things. Find out how you can help them out.

Think ahead: anticipate your partner's needs, help free up your medics hands. Be "Johnny on the spot". Communicate: talk through what you are doing. Verbalize all your moves. Know your job and the jobs around you. Set your limits/boundaries and stick to them. You're a professional, I may ask you to do things you shouldn't on accident or out of laziness or habit, it's up to you to hold your ground, don't take it personal. You never know what your partner has been through or is going through. The burn out will come, but it's up to you to fight it. Have fun with the overtime, but it's really not worth it, live within your means. Always smile."

– Chris Houston (EMT / Paramedic) 12 years experience.

"First thing, always be nice to the patient and family. The main reason EMS gets sued is because the patient/family feels disrespected or that their needs didn't matter"
– TC Warford (EMT / Paramedic) 14 years experience.

"First thing I would want them to be is comfortable and not stress about the what-if's. Be an independent thinker and think of your next move, instead of being a robot and waiting to be told to do something. Always be ahead of things. Be comfortable with each piece of equipment and knowing where it is at so when asked, you can just grab it. Lastly, know the area and where they are in relationship to the call. Stop using GPS and learn how to read a map book!"
– Brian Green (Fire Fighter / Paramedic) 24 years experience.

"MY FINAL THOUGHTS AND WORDS OF ENCOURAGEMENT"

I would like to end this book by saying accept the challenge before you. You are reading this book because perhaps you think that maybe, just maybe you can become an EMT and eventually a Paramedic, Firefighter, Nurse, P.A or even a Doctor. It doesn't matter your age or what kind of experience you have in EMS you can do this job. Many people say they could never handle all the gory parts of the job. Well I can honestly say no one can. Go on and take that EMT course! Don't wait any longer! For the new guy or gal fresh out of school....congratulations!!! Now get out there and get a job! You have all the necessary skills needed to do the job! Will it be easy at first? No. But it gets easier and easier every single day. You will become a pro in no time. We in EMS are constantly learning and this job keeps us very humble. Thank you for reading and I hope to see you in the field someday. Stay tuned for the next book in this series Fresh out of EMT school called "BLS LIFE"

God Bless You,
Albert Reyes
EMT 16 years experience

CPSIA information can be obtained
at www.ICGtesting.com
Printed in the USA
BVOW11s1754050517

483061BV00006B/117/P

9 781499 902853